Six Blue Ducks

By

Christopher C. Baker, MD

Copyright 2014 by Christopher C. Baker, M.D.

All rights reserved

ISBN-13: 978-1495278884

ISBN-10: 1495278883

Table of Contents

1. The Three A's of Success
2. Balance
3. Cleistogamy
4. The Four D's
5. Evidence Based medicine
6. Focus
7. Goal Setting
8. Humility
9. Insight and Innovation
10. Judgement
11. Knowledge Base
12. Lateral Thinking
13. Magic of Conflict
14. Neophyte
15. Observation
16. Parsimonious
17. Qualitology
18. Resourcefulness
19. Safety
20. Thixotropy
21. Understanding Others
22. Versimilitude
23. Wide Angle View
24. Xenophilia
25. Youthfulness
26. Zen

INTRODUCTION

This book is a collection of insights and aphorisms. Each chapter keys on a letter of the alphabet and has a self-contained message. One of the main themes centers on learning how to succeed in medicine and life.

This book is a tribute to my parents. My father was a general surgeon who practiced most of his career in central New Hampshire. He showed me what a life in surgery was like, how important it was to care for patients, and how to maintain a work-life balance. My mother had been an operating room nurse and was an independent soul who taught me about integrity and the importance of maintaining a sense of humor as we face the challenges in life.

You may ask about the title of this book. It stems from an experience I had in the first grade. We used mimeographed sheets to teach us numbers. One day I was faced with a sheet showing six ducks. We were supposed to color the ducks and list the number. I wrote the number "6" at the top of the page and proceeded to color the ducks blue. The teacher marked a big X on my paper because of my color choice. When I showed my mother the paper with a tear in my eye, she became furious. "This is what is wrong with education in America," she said. Her point was that education should be about understanding principles and problem solving rather than nitpicking about details. It was an important lesson, which I have carried with me to this day.

Chapter 1
The Three A's of Success

AVAILABILTY

AFFABILITY and

ABILITY in that order

If you're not available to help patients and colleagues,

If you're not easy to get along with,

Then it doesn't matter how much ability you have, you won't succeed.

Chapter 2   BALANCE

Medicine is an unforgiving mistress and will consume you if you allow it to do so. Maintaining a work-life **balance** is critical to preserving your physical and mental health.

Make it a priority to devote time to family and friends. Set limits at the hospital—it will still be there tomorrow.

I was once talking with a mentor after we had to tell a family that their son had died. As we walked away, he said "You know every time that you have to do that, it takes a piece out of you and you only have so many pieces to give."

My corollary to this is that we need to find ways to rebuild the pieces of ourselves in between times of stress.

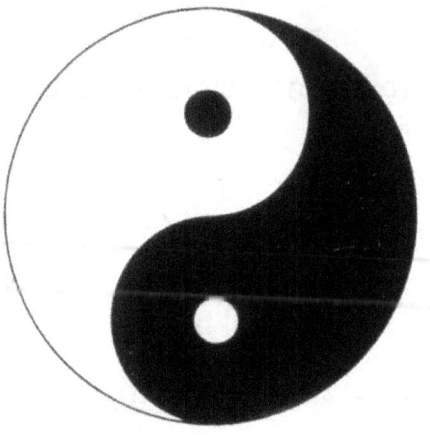

s

Chapter 3
CLEISTOGAMY

This wonderful word is a plant biology term that literally means cross-pollination.

I like to think of **cleistogamy** as the situation in which two disparate species land near each other, cross-fertilize, and produce something more beautiful and more productive than either one could make alone.

The quintessential example of this in medicine is when multidisciplinary teams work together to achieve success.

Chapter 4
The Four D's

Strive to maintain patient **dignity** at all costs.

Exercise **diligence** and attention to **detail** in all aspects of patient care.

A key precept of leadership is learning how to set priorities and **delegate.**

Learn to trust your colleagues and don't be afraid to ask for help or advice.

Chapter 5
Evidence-based Medicine

Evidence-based medicine (EBM) has been the byword for modern residency training programs. It is ideal if one can quote prospective randomized clinical trials, but they are expensive and time-consuming. Case control studies can be a reasonable compromise.

Remember the adage about "lies, damned lies and statistics."

Don't forget to recognize the difference between statistical significance and clinical significance.

Although EBM may be the gold standard, there is still a place in the clinician's database for remembering index cases that offer profound lessons.

Chapter 6 Focus

Errors tend to occur when people get distracted, whether it's behind the wheel of a car or in the operating room.

The key to success is to have a plan, to communicate the plan to the team, and to **focus** on carrying out the steps of the plan.

I can remember the feeling I had after completing a long hard operation—it was the way I felt after driving two hours in a snowstorm. The release that one feels is the result of single-minded focus on a task.

Focus requires attention to detail and devotion to the task at hand.

Chapter 7
Goal Setting

Travelling through life without **goals** is like bobbing in the ocean in a rowboat without a compass.

I once heard a speaker who asked us to make a list of 10 goals (personal and professional) for the next year. When he finished, he told us that by making a list of goals we were ahead of 90% of the population. If we actually looked at the list, we would be ahead of 95% of people. Finally, if we accomplished the goals on the list, we would be ahead of 99% of people.

One of his audience members called him up after 6 months and said he had done all the things on his list. "What do I do now," he asked. The speaker replied "Make a new list!

Chapter 8
Humility

"The only reasonable attitude for the seeker of the truth is true humility."
Bradford Cannon (1871—1945)

Medicine puts us in a position of power over patients. With this power comes great responsibility. As we care for our patients, we must avoid the twin evils of pride and arrogance.

We must maintain **humility** in the face of the trust that patients place in us. It is humility that reminds us that we will make mistakes, and it helps us learn from those mistakes. It is humility that shows us the healing power of the human soul.

As Ambrose Pare (1517-1590) said, "I dressed him, and God healed him."

Chapter 9
Insight/Innovation

Much of western thought proceeds in a vertical fashion, yet many great **insights** and **innovations** have come from lateral thinking—that process by which we shift our focus to a different organizational construct and think "outside the box."

As Louis Pasteur (1822-1895) once said, "chance only favors the prepared mind."

How many times has serendipity lead to a great discovery? Consider Fleming's experience with penicillin.

We must be open to the insights gained from pattern recognition, much as we solve a difficult problem in differential diagnosis.

Chapter 10
Judgement

We have an aphorism in surgery that "good judgement comes from experience, and experience comes from BAD judgement.

As Hippocrates (460-377 B.C.) said: "Life is short and the art long, the occasion fleeting, experience fallacious, and judgement difficult."

Cultivating excellent clinical **judgemen**t requires constant vigilance, testing of hypotheses, celebrating one's diagnostic successes, and learning from one's management errors.

The mind of the experienced clinician is a database filled with numerous individual cases that he can access to bring to bear on the clinical problem at hand.

Chapter 11
Knowledge

"Nothing is known in our profession by guess...it is right, therefore, that those who are studying our profession should be aware that there is no short road to knowledge." Sir Astley Pasten Cooper (1768-1841

The explosion of **knowledge** in the last twenty-five years has been exponential. Fortunately we have resources like the internet to help us access and categorize knowledge. Accumulation of knowledge requires the physician to be a life-long learner.

The medical student may have numerous bits of knowledge on hand, but it takes years of clinical practice to organize one's knowledge and to bring it to bear on clinical problems.

Chapter 12   Loyalty

"Few virtues are nobler than loyalty to a great tradition."
Sir Berkeley Moynihan (1865-1936)

One of the things that makes medicine a great tradition is the **loyalty** of the physician to his patients. Medicine is a great tradition because of its continual efforts to expand knowledge and improve patient care.

The physician must be loyal to the Hippocratic oath, to his patients, and to his students, residents, and colleagues. He must also remain loyal to the spirit of scientific inquiry.

Central to the concept of loyalty is the spirit of integrity, which should temper the physician's actions in every facet of life.

Chapter 13
Magic of Conflict

Conflict is inevitable in the high-stress crucible of medicine.

The title for this chapter comes from a book by Thomas Crum, an aikido master who focused on diverting the opponent's energy rather using force to resolve conflict.

In the medical setting one must remain calm and quiet, absorbing the negative energy in the situation and turning it into a positive growth experience, converting the conflict into a win-win experience. Don't have arguments in the chart and avoid heated discussions in public places.

Chapter 14
Neophytes

"If your mind is empty, it is always open to everything. In the beginner's mind there are many possibilities, but in the expert's there are few." Shunryu Suzuki (1904-1971) in <u>Zen Mind, Beginner's Mind.</u>

Teaching **neophytes** can be a challenge. I like to think of the four phases of learning:

(1) Unconscious incompetence
(2) Conscious incompetence
(3) Conscious competence
(4) Unconscious competence

For the expert (Level 4) to be a good and effective teacher, he must go back to Level 1 in his mind to remember the steps he had to take to learn as a neophyte.

Chapter 15
Observation

"You can observe a lot by watching." Yogi Berra (1925-)

Powers of **observation** are critical to being a good physician and diagnostician. Observing involves so many things:

Eye contact—looking at the patient to see what they are feeling;

Ear contact—listening to the patient for they will often give you critical clues as to what's wrong with them;

Picking up on non-verbal cues;

Identifying key physical findings; and

Using pattern recognition skills to put the whole clinical picture together.

Be open to multiple possible explanations to arrive at a cohesive diagnosis.

Chapter 16
Parsimonious

Webster defines **parsimonious** as being "frugal to the point of stinginess." What does this have to do with medicine?

When you are faced with a large constellation of physical findings and laboratory data, you must be parsimonious in your list of diagnoses. In other words, don't make five diagnoses when one will suffice to pull the multiple findings into a coherent picture.

We should also be stingy with the number of tests we order. Before ordering a test, ask yourself this question: How will the test result change my management of the patient?

When explaining things to patients, be parsimonious with your words. Use lay terminology in a clear and concise fashion.

Chapter 27
Qualitology

Quality has become a major buzzword in medicine today. Quality is being used by the federal government as a stick in pay-for-performance initiatives. Reams of data are being generated by "qualitologists" to measure quality.

True quality involves the following:

(1) Meeting the patient's needs;
(2) Coming to a diagnosis in a timely and cost-effective manner;
(3) Focusing on what's best for the patient;
(4) Minimizing errors;
(5) Communicating with patients and families in a clear and direct manner;
(6) Correcting system errors; and
(7) Tracking and reporting outcomes

Chapter 18
Resourcefulness

When facing complex challenges in medicine, one needs to rely on one's natural resources—common sense, knowledge of physiology, pattern recognition skills, and equanimity.

In surgery we often have to make critical decisions with inadequate data under the pressure of time. **Resourcefulness** involves taking stock of the tools at your command, working with the team at your side, and keeping your eye on the goal at hand.

Innovation is the ally of resourcefulness—learning to look at each problem in a new way and solving it with whatever tools one has on hand at the time, using leadership and ingenuity.

Chapter 19   Safety

Patient **safety** is a major goal in modern medicine. In surgery, the checklist concept has had a major impact on patient safety. In the complex environment of the operating room, the time-out process forces the team to stop, focus on the patient and the operation, and recognize each team member's role in the procedure. Safety is also paramount in the complex and sometimes chaotic environment in the ICU. When so many variables are changing at a rapid rate, protocols and checklists are essential to providing safe care. One of the trends that we have recognized is the syndrome of "near misses." By analyzing such events, we can understand how to prevent them from becoming errors. Lessons can be learned to prevent errors from happening in the future.

Chapter 20
Thixotropy

Thixotropy is a physical-chemical term that describes the properties of high viscosity fluids or gels. Thixotropic fluids will liquefy when shaken but solidify when left standing. The second characteristic of these gels is that when you pass an object (e.g., a bullet) through them rapidly, the kinetic energy disperses and the object will stop. Conversely if you pass the object through slowly, it will get to the other side.

Medical institutions, particularly big academic medical centers, tend to be bureaucratic and very thixotropic. If you want to generate change in such institutions, you need to shake and agitate things slowly, much like a fine martini. This one word has helped me immensely in working on institutional change.

Chapter 21
Understanding

"Medical practice is not knitting and weaving and the labor of hands, but it must be inspired with the soul and be filled with understanding and equipped with the gift of keen observation." Maimonides (1135-1204)

Understanding is central to our ability to care for patients. We must understand their stories, be aware of their feelings about their illness, and be cognizant of their hopes and fears. In a sense, we must commune with the patient and learn to interpret their words, which will often lead to a better understanding of their problem. Similarly, when we lay out our findings and our treatment plans, we must ensure that the patient has a clear understanding of what we have told them.

Chapter 22
Versimilitude

Webster describes **verisimilitude** as "the appearance of being true or the depiction of realism." It is closely related to the word *verity*, which signifies enduring truth or wisdom.

Truthfulness is at the heart of the Hippocratic oath. We need to be true to our patients and their families, who have put their trust in us. We need to be true to the highest principles of our profession. Finally, we need to be true to ourselves. We need to recognize our foibles and admit our errors. We need to be honest with ourselves when we have misgivings or self-doubt. At the end of our careers, we need to face reality and recognize that it may be time to quit. It is far better to do so gracefully rather than to overstay our welcome.

Chapter 23
Wide angle view

Analyzing and understanding complex problems is at the heart of being a good clinician. Unfortunately patients present as puzzles, not nicely wrapped packages. Although there are many skills involved in being a good diagnostician, one of the keys is the ability to have a **wide angle view**. If one hones in on a few details too early, one may miss the big picture— much like missing the forest for the trees.

While using the wide angle view, one must also exercise the skill of pattern recognition. This is what allows skilled clinicians to come to the correct diagnosis after only a short time with the patient. They have seen similar patterns in previous patients, and they have the ability the bring this to bear on the problem at hand.

Chapter 24
Xenophilia

Xenophilia is that characteristic of being comfortable with things that are foreign to oneself. As we meet patients, we are constantly exposed to differences in gender, race, creed, ethnic background, socioeconomic status, sexual orientation, political and philosophical beliefs, language, and customs. We must embrace these differences and strive to understand how they affect our patients.

In the book <u>The Dancing Healers</u>, psychiatrist Karl Hammerschlag asks a Native American medicine man how he heals. The reply—"I can show you the steps to my dance, but you must follow your own music."

Only by accepting multiple ways of healing can we become truly effective physicians.

Chapter 25
Youthfulness

George Bernard Shaw (1856-1950) once said "Youth is a great thing. It's too bad that it's wasted on the young."

Youthfulness has an effervescent, enthusiastic quality to it. The young are not afraid to take risks or try new things. As we get older we tend to become more rigid and set in our ways. One of the reasons that I have enjoyed a career in academic surgery is because working with students and residents helps keep you young. They constantly question established dogma and push the limits of our understanding. The impetus for life-long learning in medicine is one of the things that keep us young. The need to use one's mind to incorporate the rapidly expanding knowledge base in medicine is what keeps us youthful and renews us.

Chapter 26 Zen

In some respects, this chapter should be blank. **Zen** is a philosophic discipline and way of life centered on asking questions and searching for enlightenment. As Alan Watts (1916-1973) has said "In life as in art, Zen never wastes energy in stopping to explain, it only indicates." This journey of enlightenment centers on a life-long pursuit of knowledge, much as in medicine. A Zen master teaches the initiate with riddles or *koans* such as "What is the sound of one hand clapping?" The initiate must think about the *koan* and come up with a solution on his own. Often the solution will come in a flash of insight called *zazen.* This bears strong parallels to the clinician struggling to solve a difficult diagnostic dilemma. In either case the solution resides within the mind of the practitioner.

www.ingramcontent.com/pod-product-compliance
Lightning Source LLC
Chambersburg PA
CBHW070731180526
45167CB00004B/1702